LOSING

WEIGHT

IS

NOT

EASY!!

From Fat to Flab-You-Less

(This book is not for everyone)

By Ron Lee

_____

_____

_____

_____

_____

_____

_____

_____

_____

_____

_____

Acknowledgement

This area is usually where you put all the people that have helped you in reaching your goals. So I guess I will thank the women that left me because I was too Fat. They will never admit to it but everyone knows what I mean. Also, a big thank you to all my so-called friends that I had throughout my life that called me such enduring names as skinny, slim, little guy, fatty, fatso, big man, chubbo, chubby, and so on and so on. These are the people that gave me the inspiration to lose weight and be more comfortable with myself. So to all of these wonderful individuals, you can kiss all the Fat that has fallen off my Ass. Thank you.

My love and appreciation goes to my Angel. The one that has always believed in me and has never let go even when things got rough in both our lives. Thank you my imperfectly perfect puzzle piece. You are my heart.

Before we get into this book, one thing that I want to make very clear. This is not a diet book. It may be classified that way by a book store but this is not a diet book. Diet is a four letter word that makes most of us cringe when we hear it. No one wants to be on a diet. Saying you are on a diet already puts negative thoughts in your head and none of us need more of those.

Simply put this is a lifestyle change. A change for the better. You are just remodeling your body like you would your home. When you are done it will look better and be more comfortable for you to be in and just like re-doing your home it will be something that you want to show off and let everyone see how much better it looks.

There are areas throughout this book for you to write some notes if you need to.

Index

Losing Weight Is Not Easy

(This book is not for everyone)

I am going to help some of you lose weight and save money in the next minute.

If you are looking for the next best idea that will help you burn off the fat and drop weight like never before while maintaining your same lifestyle, then I have great news for you. You are one of the people that are going to lose weight and save money right now. All you need to do is lose the weight of this book by returning it and getting your money back.

"Losing Weight Is Not Easy"

There is no magic pill or supplement. No secret formula or tricks. The weight is not going to just fall off or disappear while you sleep or watch TV. You can't eat or drink whatever you want. You can't spend your time just sitting there saying "boy, I really need to lose some weight. Well it is already the middle of the week; I will get started on Monday". That Monday will never get here.

"Take Control and Make a Decision"

Most of the people that read this book are <u>FAT</u>. You have probably tried all different kinds of diets, programs, pills, supplements, plans, or miracle cures. Some have probably even had surgery. I bet for most none of them worked and you ended up back where you were or worse. Some worked a little, others not at all. The main thing that all of these have in common is "your money". They usually start with a small investment and end up with you needing to buy equipment, supplements, clothing, subscriptions, joining websites, or entering contests. All of which takes your focus away from your weight and puts it on everything you need before you can get started. Once you have everything they say you need you could have paid for that health club membership you said you couldn't afford. After you have spent a small fortune to get started and waited to get all your stuff, your motivation has taken a hit. Then you realize how much you have spent and convince yourself that you can't afford to lose weight – it costs too much.

<u>"It Doesn't Have To Be That Complicated"</u>

Losing weight does not have to be expensive. None of that stuff is necessary. That is just your way of trying to convince yourself to get started and then putting it off.

A lot of you will say you don't have the time. Well, you made the time to get FAT. Use that same time to lose the FAT. Doing all these different programs and plans; with all of their documentation, notes, planning, writing goals and menus, or going to meetings takes time away from losing weight. You can always find a way or a reason to do nothing. That's why you are where you are at with your weight.

"Losing Weight Is Not Easy"

It is time to decide if you are going to be a person that is going to lose weight and get on with your life or be that person that just thinks about it, plans for it, and spends money on it but sits on their ASS and does nothing but procrastinate.

If you are ready to get started then let's go. The thing that is different with this book is that it is being written by a FAT man in his 40's. I have tried a lot of different ways to lose weight. I know what works and what doesn't for me. So I am going to be losing weight while I write this and along with you when you are done reading this. I used to weight 500 lbs. I was able to get down to 450lbs. but was stuck there. I began to write this book and figure out what I could do about my weight problem. On 2/7/2011 I weighed 420 lbs. I will include photos and weights in this book so you can see the changes. It is hard to read diet books or do other programs or plans because they are done by people that have already lost weight or who were never FAT to begin with. For someone who has never had to struggle with eating too much or fighting to lose weight to try and tell you how to do it is just crazy. They don't understand about trying not to eat that other plate of food or dessert. To stop drinking that pop or eating that bag of chips or candy you get when you leave the store. They don't understand how easily we can justify our eating problems and then we feel bad for doing it. For some eating is a stress reliever or a comforter. For some it's because you're bored or you figure why bother nothing works. Other's do it because they are depressed or it is just a habit and we don't even think about it. You have to decide how bad you want it and what you will give up to get it. The big thing to remember is that losing weight is not easy. It is very hard, at times even painful. You have to know you will mess up or want to quit. That's ok. That's normal. Your mind and body will do things to make it hard, to make you quit. Don't give up. Every day you do well you will feel better about yourself. When you mess up and you will, you will feel bad; so what. You have felt bad for a long time now and the only one that can change that is you. Nothing is saying you can't try again. You can't change what happened or what you did so don't dwell on it. Move on.

You are probably thinking it is weird to listen to a fat man talk about how to lose weight. I will prove to you that my ideas work. You will see it in my photos and my weight. It is 7/16/2013 and I weigh 280 lbs. that means I have lost 220 lbs. since I was at my heaviest. I have had some setbacks but since I started this I have never gained the weight back just had a few stalls in losing more. There is no one set way to lose weight. Everybody is different. Some things will have to be tweaked a little for each person, but the principles are the same. Here is my email address so you can contact me and ask questions or post comments. Rattack69@hotmail.com. There is no membership fee or subscription to buy. I have nothing that you must buy or that I must sell you. I will have things that made it easier for me but there is always different ways to do things that won't cost you money. Sometimes buying things you need is easier but is in no way mandatory for my ideas to work. It is more of a convenience issue. This is not a follow along step by step approach where you can only eat this and you have to do that. The more you put into it, the faster you will see results, but that is not to say less is bad. If slower works for you then that is the best approach for you to accomplish what you want. The thing to do is listen to what has worked for me, and then try to make it your own. Remember to stay within the principal of the ideas that worked. Everyone is smart enough to know what I mean. If you think to yourself that it is wrong or not in the spirit of the meaning, then it probably is. Cheating yourself will only discourage you; so stay true to yourself.

The things that have worked for me are:

-A very strict calorie intake.

- Giving myself 1 free day a week.

- Drinking lots of water.

- Using a thermogenic product.

- Exercising every day.

- Getting plenty of rest.

I know this sounds like all the rest of them; diet, exercise, supplements. There is a difference. My way works. Everything I have tried before just sent me on a rollercoaster ride and left me worse than when I started. Everyone gives you too much to do all at once and expects you to be in good enough shape to do what they say. My way is simple and gradual so your body and more importantly your mind can adjust at a pace that won't make you give up like you have every other time. There are no crazy, spleen busting, workouts that leave you in a heap on the floor gasping for air while you're trying to dial 911.

This is your journey to take. It is not a race. No matter how slow or fast you go you can still end up in the same place.

I have read a lot of diets that want you to set goals. If that works for you then by all means do it. Just remember that if you achieve a goal don't celebrate too much there is still a long way to go. On that same note, if you don't make a goal, don't beat yourself up or give up. Be proud of what you have accomplished so far. Goals can be a tricky thing, so be careful if you use them. I don't like using goals because it is just another thing that can add stress to an already stressful situation. I work as hard as I can and I am happy with what I achieved and then I have my free day, relax, and get ready for the next round. Don't stress yourself out if you use goals. Relax and start fresh each week.

I know I said "don't stress yourself out". Yeah right. I mean don't add additional stress where you don't need to. So many Doctors, diet books, and people say that you need to reduce your stress level. Fact of the matter is, life is stressful. There is no way not to be stressed in today's world and people that are bigger (FAT) like ourselves have that as an added stress that others don't understand. Going out to eat and trying to fit in a booth and praying that they have table and chairs available, going to the movies and hoping you fit in the seats, going to places that have turn styles and trying to get through it without getting stuck and just everyday situations where you feel everyone is looking at you and making you uncomfortable. There is not a whole lot you can do about these kind of things until you start feeling better about yourself. You just have to tell yourself that you are going to lose weight and as you do you will start to feel better about yourself and have more confidence. You need to start by having the desire to lose weight and change your life. Then you need to put your desire into action and actually start doing it. The more you do it the easier it will become and the longer you do it the more it will improve your self-image and start changing your bad habits into good ones. Don't worry about everyone else. The only person you need to impress or answer to is yourself. Ultimately the only one that can change you or help you -- is you. Others can be there for support but other people can't make you want to change. The key to all of this is you and your desire to make a change.

_____

_____

_____

_____

_____

_____

_____

_____

_____

_____

_____

_____

_____

_____

_____

_____

_____

_____

Calorie Intake

(How low can you go?)

One of the biggest problems I have is that I Love Food!! The better it tastes the more I want, rather I am full or not. It is impossible for me not to clean my plate or go back for seconds or thirds or ----, just because I am full. I don't do well with diets that tell me to watch my portion size – not happening! If you have that much will power than more power to you. But how has that been working for you so far. That's what I thought. You need to figure out what your dietary intake needs to be. Mine is extremely low. I only eat between 800 to 1200 calories a day and I eat the same thing every day except my free day. I have changed my menu a couple times over the past couple years. My first menu was 2 – 90 calorie granola bars for breakfast, 1 – 310 calorie protein bar (not meal replacement bar) for lunch, and 2 – 200 calorie turkey wraps for dinner. My next menu was 1 – 900 calorie sub from subway (same sub every day) and 1 cookie. That's it. Sounds boring don't it?

That's why I do it this way. I try to teach myself not to love food. That way food does not control my life or my body. I try not to like food. Sounds extreme doesn't it, but weighing over 450 lbs. is extreme and causes the need for some drastic tactics. If you can't figure how to control your food intake then it is going to control you for the rest of your life. Think about your kids, spouse, girlfriend, best friend, etc. and how you can't play with them or run around with them or are too embarrassed to go out in public with them and then you tell me which is the extreme and which is not. Food has been our enemy for a long time.

"It's Time to Take Back Control"

When you get started, start with reduced calorie meals until you can work yourself down to what you can tolerate. You only need enough food to keep your body functioning. You don't need it because it tastes good. It won't be easy or enjoyable. Maybe you will realize just how much of a grip that food has on your life. I told you at the beginning that losing weight was not easy. Now you will start to understand and realize that this sucks. But once you get used to it you will discover that you feel better and that you are in control and that will make you work even harder. One of my biggest weaknesses was pop, Mt. Dew to be exact. I drank up to 3 – 2 liters a day. That is a lot of sugar and caffeine. This also made me crave sweets. Candy bars and pop where a very hard thing for me to get over. I was tired and had headaches. It took a couple of weeks for it to completely go away but I felt better. No more sugar roller coaster rides all day. I slept better and woke more refreshed. Getting away from these was key for me to take back control of my food problem. I could put a lot of pages of calorie charts in this book but all that would do is take up space. The best place to look up calorie charts is on the internet. You should look up some of your favorite foods and see how many calories is in some of that stuff. You will be amazed, I know I was. I will tell you that some fast food burgers have over 900 calories just for one sandwich and some complete meals at a restaurant are close to 2000 calories. Like I said before, the thing that worked best for me was to find just a couple things I could eat that would taste good and keep my calorie intake down and not eat all kinds of different foods.

You have to learn to not love food so much. Calorie intake is one of the most important things to get under control. It won't matter how much exercise you do if you can't get your calories down. Food is your enemy.

Hopefully this information will help you make better decisions and help you understand your food choices a little more. It is amazing how many calories are in some of our favorite foods, especially our fast food choices and just look at the calorie totals on some of those complete meals. It's no wonder we are so FAT.

When you are looking at the nutrition chart on the back of a food or drink item, pay close attention to how many servings are in it. I was looking at a popular sports drink the other day and a 32 oz. bottle had 50 calories on the chart and then I noticed that there were 4 servings in the bottle and all the nutritional information was per serving. So that meant I had to multiply everything by 4. That means the bottle had 200 calories in it. Also, just because an item says low fat, reduce calorie, diet, or some other labeling that makes it appear better for you doesn't mean it is. Be very careful. A lot of times these labels are very misleading; i.e.: Just because an item says low fat or even no fat doesn't mean its ok. It could have a 1000 calories worth of carbohydrates in it. A lot of products try to hook you in with such statements. Just use common sense and pay attention. Don't take their word for it; check it out. Always remember that you are in control now. This is another reason why I stick to a simple menu. These put too much time and focus back on food and caused me to think about food all day which is the opposite of what I wanted.

I have worked my way down to one meal a day. I did this pretty early on in my plan to lose weight. I know you always hear that you need to eat 5-6 small meals a day but that just does not work for me. All's that does is make me hungry all day. Eating multiple small meals throughout the day is great if you are a body builder or fitness person but we are not. We are people trying to lose weight because we are Fat. Once you get down to a weight that lets you become an active person then you can worry about maintaining energy stores for you to use but until then you have

plenty of areas where your body can feed off
of.

_____

_____

_____

_____

_____

_____

_____

_____

_____

_____

_____

_____

_____

_____

_____

_____

_____

_____

_____

_____

_____

Water Intake

(Time to know what a water balloon feels like)

Water intake is a huge part of what I do. I drink between 1 and 1 ½ gallons of water every day. Yes, that is a lot of water and it is not easy to get used to. Yes, I have to go to the bathroom a lot – a lot. Since I quit drinking pop, started exercising, and reduced my food intake it helps keep me hydrated and helps me when I start to feel hungry. Flavored water is ok as long as it is not loaded with sugars or sweeteners. The more you can stay away from colored liquids the better it will be for you. I know getting away from pop or coffee sounds impossible to some but remember I said losing weight was not easy. There are a lot of benefits to drinking water.

I have noticed a lot of benefits from drinking water. I use water to help me when I get hungry. I drink a glass of water and it helps curb my hunger feeling until I am ready to eat. It will take some time for you to get used to not eating every time you get hungry. I mean that's what we always did. That why we have the problem with food that we have. Water also gives me energy. I stopped drinking pop and replaced it with water and feel so much better now. This was very difficult for me to do but I knew it was a very important part of my plan. I felt lighter and not so full and weighted down like I felt when I was drinking pop. Plus my energy level stayed steady without having the sugar spikes and drops. My skin looks better and I don't have so many breakouts. Once I replaced my pop with water and got past the caffeine withdrawal I noticed that I started sleeping better and that has been a great help in my ability to be ready to start again the next day.

My doctor, Dr. Jones, informed me of some of the other benefits of drinking more water. Water helps increase your metabolism which helps burn fat. Drinking more water will help flush out your system by removing toxins and fat. Helps muscles from cramping, reduces headaches, regulates body temperature, prevents dehydration, eases joint pain by keeping them lubricated, aids in the digestive process so you don't get constipated, helps oxygenate your blood, and believe it or not will help you retain less water because your body doesn't think it is going to dehydrate and holds onto every drop you have. Go online and look up all the benefits that water can do for you.

_____

_____

_____

_____

_____

_____

_____

_____

_____

_____

_____

_____

_____

_____

_____

_____

_____

Think About This

(I am not going to be gentle here)

How bad do you want it? Are you in control of your life or are your habits in control of you? Are you an ADDICT?? Do your food and beverages choices give you your fix? You might know someone who is addicted to drugs or alcohol and you can't understand why they don't stop. Well, here it is. Go look in the mirror. What do you see? It's an ADDICT!! Your choice of what is destroying your body and your life is just a fix of a different nature. Sound too harsh? Does it make you mad? Too bad! You are the one that has lost control of using common sense. Don't be mad, don't be upset, and don't feel sorry for yourself. Just Get Started!! Making good decisions about hard choices will make you feel better about yourself and improve your attitude.

Is it going to be hard?   Yes.

Are you going to mess up?   Yes.

Are you going to get discouraged?   Yes.

Are you going to get mad?   Yes.

<u>SO WHAT!!</u>

Are you going to give up and have no control over your life? Are you going to let your addiction destroy your life?

<u>HELL NO!!</u>

It's time to quit coming up with reasons and excuses not to take back control. Time is running out. I believe everyone is capable of doing this. Believe in yourself or no one else will. You will doubt yourself from time to time but never give up. When you fall down you always get back up. This is the same thing. When you mess up, just start again and keep starting again until you mess up less and less.

Exercise Time

(YUK!!)

Now let's talk about exercise. Sounds like a four letter word. It is very important to start at your own pace or you will burn out to fast and give up. Obviously the harder you work out the more FAT you will burn. Don't push yourself so hard that you are miserable but if you are not uncomfortable then you are wasting your time. Don't try to keep up with someone else, you probably won't be able to at first. You don't need all kinds of equipment or memberships. All you need is a pair of comfortable walking shoes and a stopwatch or timer of some sort. Determine how far you can walk in a certain period of time. Such as, walk for 10 minutes then turn around and walk back. As time goes by you will be able to make that same trip a little faster. That's when it is time to walk a little further. When you exercise, whether you are walking, riding a bike, or using cardio equipment it is important to speed up and slow down during your routine. Go for 2 minutes at a good pace then do a 30 second burst then 2 minutes and so on. This will help burn FAT long after you are done exercising. *Remember to stay hydrated*. When you first get started only do what you are capable of. Maybe you can only walk to the end of your driveway and back or even to your front door and then back to your chair. Anything is better than nothing. You just need to get going. You can increase your distance and time as you get in better shape. Don't get too comfortable in your routine; always try to push a little more. I know what you're thinking – this really sucks. Well guess what – being FAT sucks even more. If you are fortunate enough to have exercise equipment or a gym membership, all the better, it will just make it easier to have different choices but don't think they are mandatory or necessary, just helpful. Once you work yourself up to it, a good cardio routine will last 30 to 40 minutes. Even little extra things like parking further away from an entrance or taking the stairs instead of an elevator. Even if you can only do 1 flight of stairs and then take the elevator the rest of the way and the same coming back down, every little bit helps.

Here is a list of exercises that will help. Are you ready?

 Walking. That's it. I could give you hundreds of exercises that would help you lose weight and tighten and tone your body but I don't think that would help because you have not done them yet. Walking is simple to do. There are no special instructions, just one foot in front of the other then repeat. Keep repeating until you're not FAT. The point is, if you can't walk very far or very fast the other exercises won't do you any good at this point. Once you can walk a couple miles without needing an oxygen tank to help you breath is when you can start looking at other exercises you can try. It is important to keep it simple when you start. Too many things at once can be overwhelming and people like us don't need any more reasons not to try.

It is important to do a little every day because if not, it is just that much easier to put it off until another day. Then before you know it a week has gone by. You need to make exercise a habit. It is always good to replace bad habits like eating with good habits like exercising. Also the more you exercise the less you will want to eat bad food because you will not want to have done all that work just to waste it on a bad meal or snack. Try to incorporate or at least inform friends and family of what you are doing so they can be supportive and not cause any unnecessary temptation. As crazy as it sounds, you will start having more energy throughout the day and sleep better at night, just from exercising. Exercising and staying hydrated will help with all sorts of bodily functions, appearance, and behavior. If you are having a rough day or getting really stressed out, a little exercise will clear your head and elevate your mood. Then things won't look so bad and you can work on things with a clear head. Stop being the victim of your addiction and take back control of your life. Once you are in control you will have more confidence and that is something no one can take away from you because it is yours and you made it happen.

_____

_____

_____

_____

_____

Time for a Free Day

(HURRAY)

I know you've been waiting for this part. A free day is just what it sounds like. A day for you to relax, sit around, eat deliciously crappy food, and take a break from the Hell of losing weight. Enjoy but don't overdo it because you can make yourself sick with all that food. On this day don't worry about your plan to lose weight. This day is to help you reset so you can get back in the battle tomorrow. As you lose weight and start feeling better and having more energy you can use this day to do more things with your friends and family. Remember only 1 free day a week. That means 6 days working on your weight problem and then a free day then 6 days and so on. Free days are not to be back to back because that means you will have to go to long before you get another one and that will really screw you up. I actually think about my free day during the week to give me motivation to make it to that day. Eventually your free day won't be that big of a deal and you won't plan how much crap you're going to eat on that day. I know you think I am full of it now but trust me; this is the natural progression of how this works. It gets easier I promise.

Here's Something to Think About

Have you ever noticed how important food is in our everyday life? Everything we do is surrounded by food. Everywhere you go, everything you see on TV is surrounded by food. There are advertisements, commercials, samples, give aways, coupons, and smells pumped out of restaurants to get your attention. Almost every event has to have food; weddings, funerals, holidays, birthdays, anniversaries, sports events, shopping, and celebrations of any kind always seems to involve food. This makes things very hard for FAT people because food is what makes us comfortable, and then we get a big plate of food and feel uncomfortable because we think everyone is looking at us. Kind of a vicious cycle isn't it. You need to stop loving food, it's not worth it. This will not be easy. This will not be fun. This will be hard. Suck it up and take control. You are not a victim. You are an addict. Quit blaming everything else. This is your fault. This is your problem and this will be your Victory. You can do this --- trust me. Now get out there and push yourself a little harder.

_____

_____

_____

_____

_____

_____

_____

_____

_____

_____

_____

_____

_____

_____

_____

_____

_____

_____

zzz Rest zzzz

(Work hard enough to deserve this)

Oh yeah!! After some of your days you are going to love your bed. This is not a complicated part of what you need to do. Sleep is a vital part of this working. Don't be surprised if at times you have a hard time getting to sleep. You are going to be sore. Your legs are going to ache and you may even get some cramps at first. If you have this problem a hot shower or soaking in the tub before you go to bed will help a lot. Staying hydrated will help with cramping along with different supplements which I will get into later. If you're worn out – rest. If you're tired – sleep. If you're hurting – good job. Keep it up. Don't abuse this part; too much sleep will actually take away a lot of your energy. Use common sense. If you stay in bed you are not going to lose weight. There will be days when it hurts to get up. This is because your body is using muscles it forgot it had and probably wished it had gotten rid of. You will be sore. It's ok. As long as you exercise within your limits you will be fine. You will be sore but fine and it's ok to curse at me I can't hear you. Just don't stop.

Getting to proper amount of rest is vital to losing weight along with other body functions. Proper sleep will help reduce your stress levels which you are going to need after a day of looking at all that chocolate that you can't eat. You can look but do not touch. Your aching swollen feet, ankle, legs, etc. are going to appreciate the rest. They will actually start repairing themselves and the swelling you are going to encounter will go down. Sleep helps will memory issues and depression which I am sure some of you have because of how much you weigh. There are a lot more benefits to proper rest so I encourage to find out more so you will understand how important this part is.

_____

_____

_____

_____

_____

_____

_____

_____

Supplements

Supplements are boring, not mandatory, and some taste terrible but they are helpful, easy to use, and can make you feel better. The best supplement you can use is a good quality multi-vitamin. With the reduction in your food intake a good vitamin can help out a lot. Supplements can be very confusing with all the ads about what you need and what the next miracle item is. Most of these are just fluff to get your money. I will discuss the basics of what will be helpful. None of us reading this book are going to be body builders or fitness instructors so we don't need to understand all there is to know about all the different supplements. So here is a list of the basic supplements I have used.

Vitamins. If you are going to choose any of these chose this one first. Vitamins are very important to proper body function. Since you are going to be changing what you eat it would be a good idea to take a good multi-vitamin. Not a cheap bottom of the barrel vitamin but a good quality vitamin from a health food store. The biggest difference in vitamins is how well they are absorbed into the body if you buy a crappy vitamin you're going to get crappy results from it.

Thermogenic. I use these on a regular basis because they seem to help me. Rather it helps for real or just mentally, I get better results when I use them. There are many different brands that you can try. My best advice is to ask around and research it for yourself so you can find the one that meets your requirements because everyone is different. What works for me might not work for you.

Protein. Whey or Casein protein is a good way to help your body heal. It is a good thing to take at night as a snack if you need one. It will assist in repairing your body while you sleep.

There are a ton of different types of supplements and just as many opinions about them. The ones I told you about are the basics and anything beyond these is not very important at this point. Don't let a supplement shop talk you into a bunch of stuff you don't need. None of this is mandatory. The amount of money you spend is not going to determine how much weight you lose. You don't have to spend a dime to lose weight. You just have to get up and start doing something, anything, just stop doing nothing.

_____

_____

_____

_____

_____

_____

_____

_____

_____

_____

_____

_____

_____

_____

_____

_____

_____

_____

_____

Helpful Items

The key word here is helpful. Nothing on this list is mandatory. Weight loss is not a matter of how much money you have or how many things you can buy. Everything you need to lose weight has already been built into your body. The only thing that is mandatory is a brain. If you don't have one of those then you haven't made it this far into the book and I don't have to worry about hurting your feelings. You can have almost any kind of disability and still be able to do this. Anyone can find an excuse not to try. Remember these are just things that can help make it a little easier but you will do just fine without them. So here we go. A pair of walking shoes; although not mandatory, these are probably the most helpful item you could have. Your feet will thank you. A picture of yourself before you get started so you can compare it to yourself later. I know horrifying thought. You don't have to show anyone, this is just for you. It helped me. Granted I needed a wide angle panoramic camera for my first picture. (Ha Ha). A scale will help you track your weight loss. Don't worry if you have an old scale the dial will quit spinning. A blender for mixing shakes. A water bottle to take with you when you walk or go somewhere, so you don't stop and buy a pop. Baby powder or talc to apply to areas that are chaffing from the friction caused by working out. Ice pack or heating pad for sore muscles. Blister prevention socks or blister pads because you will probably get some once you start walking a lot. See, all very simple. You are the main thing - not stuff. No need for a second mortgage to buy things. Like I said these are just suggestions to make it easier. Remember everyone is different and different things will work for different people. This is not a cookie cutter plan. This is a completely customizable plan tailored to fit anybody that wants to put in the effort.

_____

_____

_____

_____

_____

_____

_____

_____

Warning Signs

I am going to go over some basic warning signs you could encounter while trying to lose weight. This is not a complete list of warning signs. If you experience problems or have concerns you need to contact your doctor immediately or go to the emergency room or call 911. You know your body better than anyone so if you're having a problem get immediate help. Use common sense. Not that difficult. So here are some warning sign or symptoms:

Cramps – This will happen from over doing it and getting dehydrated.

Muscle soreness – This will most likely happen. If the soreness is painful seek medical attention if you think it is beyond what you think is normal for what you have done.

Chest pains – Stop. Get help immediately.

Bruising

Excessive swelling – Some is normal but don't let it get to bad. My feet would swell up all the time until I got used to all the walking I was doing.

Any other conditions that causes you concern should be dealt with before it gets too bad. If you think it is a concern have it checked out because it is going to take your focus away from what you are working on until you have it dealt with.

Ok, that's it. Now it's time to get started. Not tomorrow. Not next week. Right now. Oh crap, you mean right now don't you? Yes, I mean right now. How much longer are you going to keep coming up with an excuse to stay FAT? Did you think that just because you bought the book that I was going to reveal some miracle way to hold this book while I erased your FAT away magically? I gave you fair warning at the beginning that this was no miracle cure. This is hard work but you can do it. What have you got to lose just by giving it a try? Oh yeah, years of built up FAT. Now get off your Butt and get going. Take control back.

<u>You Can Do This!!!</u>

We need to record some personal information to help track how you are doing. It is pretty self-explanatory. This information is just for you. No one else has to see these. Once a month fill in the next chart and see how you have done from the previous month or from where you started. Keep notes if that works for you. When you weigh yourself, do it at the same time in the morning to get a consistent reading.

_____

_____

_____

_____

_____

_____

_____

_____

_____

_____

_____

_____

_____

_____

_____

_____

Now we need to get some stats.

Start Date: _____

Height: _____ Weight: _____

Pant size: _____ Shirt Size: _____

Measurements

Neck	
Chest	
Abdomen	
Waist	
Left Thigh	
Right Thigh	
Left Arm	
Right Arm	

Now we need to get some stats.

Date: _____

Height: _____ Weight: _____

Pant size: _____ Shirt Size: _____

Measurements

Neck	
Chest	
Abdomen	
Waist	
Left Thigh	
Right Thigh	
Left Arm	
Right Arm	

Now we need to get some stats.

Date: _____

Height: _____ Weight: _____

Pant size: _____ Shirt Size: _____

Measurements

Neck	
Chest	
Abdomen	
Waist	
Left Thigh	
Right Thigh	
Left Arm	
Right Arm	

Now we need to get some stats.

Date: _____

Height: _____ Weight: _____

Pant size: _____ Shirt Size: _____

Measurements

Neck	
Chest	
Abdomen	
Waist	
Left Thigh	
Right Thigh	
Left Arm	
Right Arm	

Now we need to get some stats.

Date: _____

Height: _____ Weight: _____

Pant size: _____ Shirt Size: _____

Measurements

Neck	
Chest	
Abdomen	
Waist	
Left Thigh	
Right Thigh	
Left Arm	
Right Arm	

Now we need to get some stats.

Date: _____

Height: _____ Weight: _____

Pant size: _____ Shirt Size: _____

Measurements

Neck	
Chest	
Abdomen	
Waist	
Left Thigh	
Right Thigh	
Left Arm	
Right Arm	

Now we need to get some stats.

Date: _____

Height: _____ Weight: _____

Pant size: _____ Shirt Size: _____

Measurements

Neck	
Chest	
Abdomen	
Waist	
Left Thigh	
Right Thigh	
Left Arm	
Right Arm	

Now we need to get some stats.

Date: _____

Height: _____ Weight: _____

Pant size: _____ Shirt Size: _____

Measurements

Neck	
Chest	
Abdomen	
Waist	
Left Thigh	
Right Thigh	
Left Arm	
Right Arm	

Notes

Notes

Notes

Notes

Pictures, Weights, & Dates

500lbs. 12/25/2008

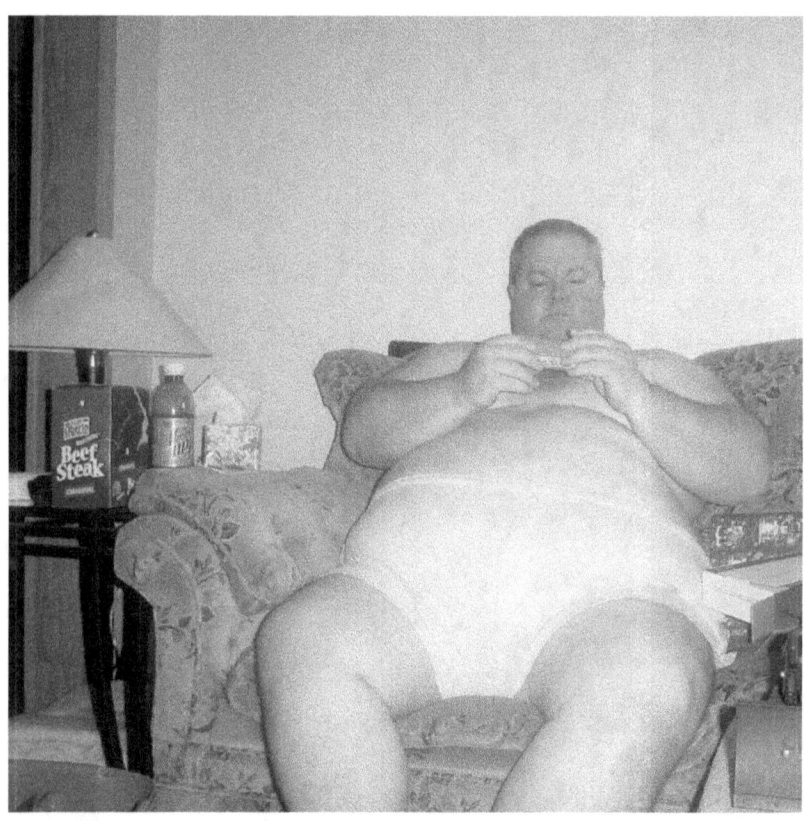

I had a hard time even getting off the couch at times. This is what I was talking about earlier. This is insane living your life like this.

490 lbs. 07/18/2009

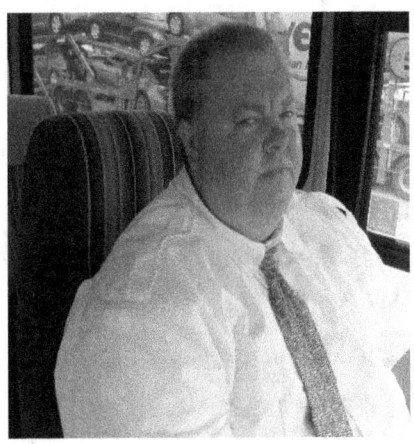

I was so big I had a hard time even sitting behind a steering wheel in most vehicles and trying to find a place to sit in a restaurant was next to impossible.

_____

_____

_____

_____

_____

_____

_____

_____

_____

_____

_____

As of the publication date of this book, on 08/03/2013, I currently weigh 280 lbs. That means I have lost 220 pounds from my heaviest weight of 500 lbs. and since I started working solely with these guidelines on 02/07/2011 at a weight of 420 lbs. I have lost 140 lbs. I have had periods of time when I didn't lose anything because of personal issues that took my focus away from what I was doing. I have never gained the weight back just stopped losing for periods of time.

I had an average weight loss of about 10 – 15 lbs. a month when I was following it properly. I made mistakes and messed up from time to time. I just picked up where I left off and kept going. I am still working on losing weight and will gladly share a picture if you want to email me at rattack69@hotmail.com.

Always remember to keep what works best for you and get rid or change what is holding you back. There is no one strict way to do this. I will be glad to offer any assistance I can by contacting me at the above email address.

280 lbs. 08/03/2013

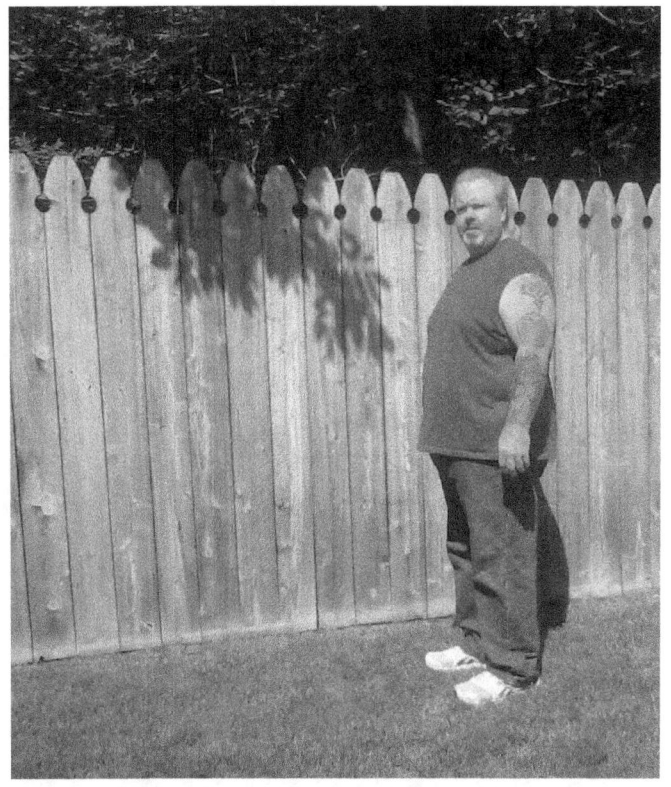

I still have more weight to lose but it will happen. You can see the difference between where I was and were I am.

Losing Weight Is Not Easy

(But it is worth it)

Good Luck!! You can do this.

www.ingramcontent.com/pod-product-compliance
Lightning Source LLC
Chambersburg PA
CBHW070822290526
45795CB00002B/808